Natural Skin Care Recipes

From a French Woman's Kitchen

Elodie Lefrancois

Elodie Lefrancois

Table of Contents

Introduction

Bonjour!

I want to thank you for purchasing, "***Skin Care Recipes from a French Woman's Kitchen.***"

I am Elodie Lefrancois, and I was born in a little village in Provence where I learned to love all the wonderful things Mother Nature has to offer. Taking long walks in the mornings with my Grand'Mere, my Maman, or my Tantes (Aunties in English), while inhaling the intoxicating aroma of the lavender fields, are some of my greatest childhood memories.

It was on these walks that I received my education about nature's beauty and how it related to my own. Grand'Mere would always carry a basket which we would fill with flowers, herbs, and medicinal plants as we walked. Sometimes my aunts or mother would join us and we would spend the entire morning together. I would run around and play, but always listen as they gathered their bounty and discussed what they would do with this particular flower, or that plant they had just found.

I had no idea they were teaching me everything I would ever need to know about nature, beauty, and the gentle arts of being a woman. These special strolls taught me the value of caring for myself and my family, being confident and beautiful in my own skin, and all of the little tricks and secrets I needed to know to enhance what Mother Nature had given me.

As a young woman, I fell in love with an American University student and packed my bags to follow my new husband back to his home in the Southern United States. Here in Virginia, I have made my home and spent most of my adult life.

I have had the honor to meet some strong and intelligent women whom I call my closest friends, and one of our favorite things to do is to take long morning walks through the countryside, often bringing our daughters, discussing the ways to use Mother Nature's bounty to better care for ourselves and our families, along with the little tricks and secrets that strengthen our spirits and add beauty to our lives.

As we walk, we will find things we can use to make a scrub, or a bath treatment, or to cure dry skin or a pimple. Through the years, my lovelies have listened to me go on and on about making this potion or that, and they have told me to write a book at least a hundred times. So finally I decided to spend the chilly winter months cozily ensconced by the fire writing a little recipe book any woman could use to make wonderful all-natural skin treatments right out of her own kitchen.

Women love to create: it is woven into our DNA. And while you and I may not be able to walk through the lavender fields in Provence or the countryside of Virginia to gather the raw ingredients, I hope you'll enjoy this little recipe book, and that it will help you create your own tailored beauty products and skin care solutions for any special issues you may have.

These recipes will not only help you look good, but feel wonderful as well. They are even more special because they are made with love and your own hands.

Before we go any further though, it is important to understand that if there is one thing a French woman knows with complete certainly, it's that beauty is an attitude. If you *feel* good, you can't help but look good. No matter what you put on the outside, whether it's expensive clothes or makeup, your confidence radiates from the inside.

A confident woman stands strong in a chaotic world and walks lightly but surely on the earth. Every woman wants to look and feel her best, no matter which continent she comes from, and beauty is understood in every language, with no translation required.

So settle in with a cup of tea or a glass of wine, and join me as we explore the beauty and bounty of Mother Nature.

Elodie

Your Kitchen of Creation

Beauty does not come from your makeup bag. That expensive collection of bottles and tubes only covers up the imperfections that you do not want the world to see- it does not make the beauty. Every perfectly polished lady knows that beauty is what shines from the inside. If you want to hide behind a costly mask, just close this book, because you will not want to hear anything else that I have to say.

You see, everything we need to look and feel our best can come right out of our kitchens. And, with a little guidance, you can learn how to specially tailor all of your beauty products specifically for you, or your family.

It is sheer joy creating your own personal care items, and it is joyous when others notice a change in you. Then you can share these gifts with your loved ones because everyone will want to know your secrets. When you think about it, as women, we are designed to be the creatures of creation. It gives us great satisfaction when we prepare a lovely holiday meal, make a home, or, most importantly, the first time we hold our children in our arms. We feel a deep sense of accomplishment when our creations result in perfection; they fill us with a great sense of belonging and purpose.

Making your own skin care and personal care products can be just as rewarding (maybe not the same as holding your child for the first time, but most certainly as rewarding as planting a garden or writing a book).

The process of creating your own products is a much more enjoyable experience when you have everything ready to use at your fingertips. Organizing all of the products and tools needed makes the experience much more fun. So, the first plan of action (after you finish this book) is to clean your kitchen and assemble all of the tools and supplies needed for your Skin Creations.

In the following chapters, we will discuss what you will need to make your products, what results you will be looking for, and of course, how to make them. So let's get started.

The first thing I want you to do is take a look at some old photographs from around the turn of the last century (you can Google a few, I'll wait…). You'll see that unless a woman worked outside in harsh conditions, she generally did not show the signs of aging as most women do in modern times. There are many reasons that older generations retained their youthful glow more than we have.

First, the water they drank was most likely *not* purified or recycled. It came fresh out of the ground; crystal clear and cold. No chemicals were used in purification and not as many toxins were running off of the roads and farm lands and into the water supply. And they certainly did not recycle and purify human waste for consumption as some modern municipalities do.

Not only did our ancestors drink better water in general, but they also grew their own food in richer soil without chemicals, hunted for or raised the livestock that they ate, and preserved food in natural ways that were not as harmful to the human body as modern processing.

Whenever you eat packaged or commercially canned food, you're consuming a veritable cocktail of man-made chemicals which the body has no idea how to break down and digest. Those foreign agents sit on the walls of our organs, veins, and arteries; and ultimately, for most, result in people who are sick, overweight, and have bad complexions.

These little tidbits of information are to increase your awareness for a lifelong path of health and beauty. Healthy aging lets us grow older gracefully while feeling fantastic as time marches on.

That said, we need to make sure we understand what it really means when we see the words "Natural", "Organic", and "Certified Organic" on products and in shops, because the differences between the three are worlds apart.

Products marked with the word "natural" can be an evil deception. The word "organic" is not much different. Most things that you buy are derived from a natural source and are somewhat organic. After all, both words simply mean something derived from nature, and in the case of "organic," something that is derived from a living organism.

In the beauty world, things like oatmeal (grains), sugar (refined sugars), and natural oils all come from a "natural" source. But, when manufactures put these natural products into a container, they are required by law to add chemical preservatives to keep the products from spoiling, "contaminating" other products, or inviting pests. That's great for public safety and preserving profit margins, but it's not necessarily in the best interest of your body.

The term "organic" can be just as deceiving. When my cat makes a deposit in the yard, it is essentially an organic substance, but it doesn't mean I'm going to eat it or rub it all over my skin! And, just like the term *natural*, products marked with the *organic* label must have pure contents, but read the packages and be wary of chemical preventives.

There *are* wholesome natural things that can be added that are not harmful, such as citric acid or ascorbic acid, which are totally acceptable. However, the best thing you can do for your good health, and radiant beauty, is to ensure you are getting the best products available. "Certified organics" go through rigid protocols and are monitored by officials that take their jobs, and your health, very seriously.

The cost for these items is a little more, but it is my belief that one can never put a price on one's health. Why would you risk compromising your health when you can take matters in your own hands?

Some things we can change, and others we have to make do with, but once you begin to take your health and beauty into your own two hands, you will never go back to buying garbage to put on, or in, your face.

So now, before you read on any further, take a pen and paper and write down a list of the beauty issues you would like to change about your skin and body in particular: everything from stress, acne, dry patches, scalp issues, or anything that is bothersome to you. Write this list from a place of confidence and possibility, not self-doubt or self-loathing. Then as you go through the rest of this book, pay particular attention to those issues first, then branch out to other texts and resources.

Now, let's get to the reason we have come together and let me share with you some of the little secrets that the women in my life once shared with me.

The Foundation of Self-Care - Aromatherapy

Like *natural* and *organic*, another word that gets thrown around and misunderstood is *aromatherapy*.

Aromatherapy is a loosely and mostly undefined description that is used commercially to describe the fragrances used in everything from air fresheners, carpet deodorizers, and candles to pretty much anything that has a "pleasing" aroma. These products can often smell okay and do a good job in covering up household odors, however, most are *loaded* with man-made chemicals and substances that are not healthy for the human body.

There's a reason so many people get an instant headache upon entering one of the popular candle shops or perfume shops. For some, even walking down the detergent aisle in the grocery store can trigger allergic reactions and blinding headaches. It's not that there's anything wrong with the person, the body simply is not designed to be assaulted with these substances.

When I use the term *aromatherapy*, I am describing more than a pretty fragrance. Aromatherapy is actually a branch of holistic medicine that uses ancient practices to prevent and treat sickness and leaves a person with a general sense of wellbeing.

Aromatherapy is defined as using plant-based extracts to improve the quality of life. Most commonly these plant-based extracts are in the form of oil called essential oils. Do not mistake essential oils as the common form of oil that you cook with, or something like baby oil, which is a heavy, greasy substance that leaves a residue behind.

Essential oils are the molecular essence of plant-based material that can penetrate human skin, enter the blood, and even cross the blood-brain barrier, whereas regular oils simply sit on top of the skin, leaving a greasy, sticky residue that can clog pores and make your skin a general mess.

The art of aromatherapy entails learning how to masterfully use essential oils to prevent and treat issues that may cause distress in the human body. These oils need to be respected as medicine and handled with care. If not used properly, they can cause some injury to skin or the mucus membranes.

They should be kept away from children and stored away from direct sunlight or extreme temperatures. Do not be frightened by these warnings! These are the wonderful gifts from Mother Nature but, remember that too much of anything, even a *good* thing, can cause harm to the body.

While we're not going to go deep into aromatherapy in this book, we will cover enough of the basics so you can begin using essential oils for yourself and to the benefit of your family.

This type of oil is obtained in many different ways, depending on the extraction method that is used for a particular plant or herb. How it is obtained is not really important unless you want to know more about a specific brand and a specific treatment.

The purest oils are Certified Organic Essential Oils, and if you need to know the exact form of distillation, you are in luck, because the beauty of the Certified Organic System is that every step is documented. This ensures the most pure ingredients that money can buy, and your body will thank you.

With the massive variety of Essential Oils on the market, it is hard to choose which to buy. For the purposes of this book, we will start with a very small list, but throughout the book I will list some optional oils you may want to experiment with later on down the line. Just remember to use a very minimal amount until you know exactly how your skin will react.

The first oils you should buy for creating your natural skin care products are Lavender, Peppermint, Lemon, Orange, Tea Tree, Chamomile, Eucalyptus, Grapefruit, Ylang-Ylang, and Geranium. Rose is also an amazing essential oil, but prepare yourself for a bit of a shock where the cost is concerned. A 5mL bottle can cost upwards of $250, but you can buy in smaller amounts and use it judiciously.

The costs of these oils are justified considering how much plant material is needed to make these amazing gifts from nature. It takes 60,000 roses to make one ounce of essential oil, and over 10,000 pounds of rose blossoms to make just 1 pound of the oil. Considering the cost of a bouquet of flowers today, you're getting a bargain with the oils.

Here is a general description of the ten oils mentioned above:

Lavender Oil

This oil mixes and blends well with almost every other essential oil. A common and well-known fragrance that brings a soothing and relaxing calm to the sprit, lavender oil can be used generously on the body and used to calm irritated skin. Lavender essential oil can be used as an insect repellent and also on bug bites and stings, so don't forget to carry it with you on outdoor excursions.

Having a small bottle of this oil in my handbag saved me a trip to the doctor when my husband and I were on a house hunting expedition. We were exploring the back yard of the home we now live in when I stepped in a massive hornet's nest. I was stung fifteen or twenty times before I was able to get away, but by applying the lavender oil immediately (after securing my person in the car!) I was able to minimize the swelling and stop the histamine reaction. Our real estate agent was stunned!

Peppermint Oil

A strong essential oil that has endless uses, peppermint oil can stimulate a tired mind and is fantastic for digestive distress and headaches. I keep a small vial of this one in my purse too for everything from chemical overload headaches at the grocery store, to the nausea associated with motion sickness when traveling.

I also mix it into my kitchen cleaners because bugs cannot stand Peppermint essential oil, plus it cuts through grease on any surface. Additionally it can be used in small amounts to soothe tired muscles, help fight acne, and is great for flu season. One drop of therapeutic grade oil can turn an ordinary cup of hot tea into a healing Peppermint Tea Tonic.

Lemon and Orange Oils

These oils are very similar, and I use them together or separately depending on what fragrance I'm looking for. I use the Orange oil to clean my appliances and furniture. I use

Lemon oil, in my iced tea and water. I also put a drop in my conditioner, or mix it with Lavender and use as a room spray. In skin care, I use them both in almost every product and Detox Bath I make to liven up my skin and brighten my mood.

Tea Tree Oil

The Essential Oil of Tea Tree is one of the strongest anti-viral substances found on the planet. I use it mainly in my cleaning products on surfaces where many use bleach: it can cut through any type of nastiness you may have and is safe for most anything that can be wet cleaned.

It is also fantastic for nail fungus and athlete's foot fungus. Tea Tree essential oil is an ideal treatment for teenage acne, blemishes, oily skin, and can be added to shampoo and conditioner to help treat scalp disorders. When using it on the skin, use it sparingly and be prepared for the strong astringent smell.

Chamomile Oil

Chamomile essential oil has a beautiful and almost romantic fragrance: one whiff will change your whole attitude. This oil can help alleviate depression and anxiety and restore a sense of hope. You can use it in a diffuser to calm fussy children (and husbands) and is great to calm very irritated skin. Chamomile is fantastic for sensitive skin and a great cure for acne.

Eucalyptus Oil

Eucalyptus essential oil is wonderful to have on hand for a variety of ailments. Use it in a diffuser to cleanse the air in the house when sinus issues and colds come to call. It's a fantastic grease-cutting cleanser that leaves a pleasant fragrance while emitting a sense of wellbeing. I use this in my bath every evening in the winter months and it is something I look forward to all day long. You can also sprinkle it on firewood a couple days before it is burned to fill the house with a bracing woodsy aroma.

Grapefruit Oil

Grapefruit essential oil refreshes, revitalizes, and awakens the skin by improving circulation. Used directly on areas affected by cellulite, it helps minimize the embarrassing lumps and bumps and improves the texture of the skin. Also, it is a great addition to detoxifying baths and to skin care for a glowing complexion. This oil is almost as essential as lipstick.

Ylang-Ylang Oil

There just aren't words to describe how magnificent the aroma of Ylang-Ylang oil is. It makes you relax into thoughts of lazy early summer evenings in the garden, and the effect that it has on the senses is sublime. It can be used alone as a sensual, romantic perfume, or in the bathtub for a relaxing, indulgent soak. Men seem to be very attracted to this fragrance, so you might want to keep this in mind for a special date night.

Add a couple of drops to your shampoo, or diffuse it with an oil diffuser to surround yourself with happiness. The options are endless and it is a very addictive fragrance, so prepare to put the cost of this oil into your monthly budget. Luckily this one is not nearly as costly as rose oil!

Rose Oil

The Essential Oil of Rose is the epitome of luxury: one drop of this magic elixir can make you feel like the most special woman in the world. It has so many uses that can be implemented into every part of your beauty regimen and wellbeing. I usually only buy one 5mL bottle a year and cherish tiny every drop. I make a bottle of perfume with this oil mixed with a bit of ylang ylang oil and only use it on very special occasions.

Treating Specific Skin Conditions

Grand'Mere used to tell me that when it comes to Nature's Bounty, whatever smells best to you, and appeals to your senses, is exactly what your body needs. When shopping for essential oils, take the time to sample the testers and listen to what your body is telling you.

Some of the most popular fragrances may not appeal to you at all, a strong indication that you do not need that one. I apply this principle to every aspect of my life and it has served me and my family very well. A woman's instinct is a force that should not be taken lightly- listen to it.

Below is a list of Essential Oils that can be used for different issues – use this as a jumping off point for exploration.

Oils to Help Eczema
- Bergamot
- Chamomile
- Lavender
- Patchouli

To Help Psoriasis
- Bergamot
- Cedarwood
- Geranium

For Dry Skin
- Sandalwood
- Ylang Ylang

- Geranium

To Treat Acne
- Basil
- Tea Tree
- Orange
- Lemon
- Orange
- Rosemary

For Fine Lines and Wrinkles
- Rose
- Geranium
- Chamomile
- Ylang Ylang
- Sandalwood

In addition to essential oils, there are number of things you will need to begin your self-made skin care journey. I suggest reading through the book to see what interests you, and taking notes. At the end of the book will be a list of additional supplies that you may want to add to your pantry.

Cleanse, Renew, and Refresh

Aesthetic beauty, the beauty that we see on the outside, all begins deep inside the body at the cellular level. When the cells in your body can perform and do their job effectively, beauty shines on the outside. We all are aware that we need to eat good food, get plenty of exercise, sufficient rest, and drink at least 8 glasses of water a day, but not many of us actually follow these guidelines. Ironically, when we stray from this we fall sick, sometimes from serious forms of disease.

Let's continue our journey by going inside and working our way to the surface, because, of course, beauty begins on the inside.

Detox

The first step in changing your outward beauty is cleaning out the toxins that have accumulated in the deep cavities of your body. The products that you put on your skin will work better if they do not have to fight deep-seated obstacles. Begin your beauty transformation with some heavy detoxing, which begins with clean water.

The body is made up of 70% water, so it is of the utmost importance to keep that water clean. You would not leave a container of water out in the garden near the compost heap for a couple of days and then drink it. But by not drinking enough good, pure water you are essentially doing just that to the water in your body. If you are not drinking an adequate amount of *clean* water, your cells are drinking *dirty* water.

Use some of the following recipes to aid in your water intake and detoxing your system.

Lemon Water

Begin every morning with 4 oz. of water mixed with the juice of half an organic lemon. This will slowly balance the pH inside the body and begin pushing the junk out. Use only organic lemons so you're not ingesting more toxins and pesticides while you're trying to "clean house."

Herbal Teas

The organs of the body are usually where disease takes hold. Make a habit of flushing the organs with herbal teas to keep them clean and functioning properly. Teas are a delicious way to ensure a beautiful complexion and ensure a long healthy life.

Try a few tea recipes that can help you remove toxins from the body and help clear up imperfections on the skin:

Ginger Root Tea
- Cut off a 1 inch section of organic ginger root
- Grate the ginger
- Put into a tea ball
- In a big mug, pour 6 oz. of boiling water over the tea ball
- Let it steep for 10 minutes
- Remove tea ball and add honey to taste

Ginger is very good for the digestive tract and will help break down the impurities that are stuck to the walls of these organs. Keeping the digestive tract free from debris is not only good for your skin; it is good for a long healthy life.

Lavender and Chamomile
- Using the sprigs from a fresh stalk of Lavender or packaged Lavender buds, fill a tea ball half full
- Using dried Chamomile petals, fill the remainder of the tea ball
- Pour 6 oz. of boiling water over the tea ball
- Steep for 10 minutes
- Remove the tea ball and add honey to taste

Lavender and/or Chamomile is very good for acne prone, irritated, or sensitive skin. Chamomile has a relaxing effect on the body and is very good to enjoy before bed.

Green Tea with Rose Hips
Rose Hips can be purchased from your natural food store, or you can use the essential oil of rose hips. If you are using the packaged version, follow the directions for the other teas above. If you want to try using the essential oil, it is just as easy:

- Boil 6 oz. of water and put into a big mug
- Add 6-10 drops of the Rose Hip Oil to taste
- Add honey as desired

Rose Hips are good for many things, and are highly recommended for dry and/or sensitive skin. Rose Hips can also help with arthritis and hot flashes.

You can use the guidelines above to come up with your own specially brewed teas. Be very careful when experimenting with teas made with essential oils because you do not want to add too much or use an oil not suitable for internal consumption. Always read the labels and understand that essential oils can cause your body to detox too quickly.

Don't be afraid though, just add 1 drop at a time and stop if you start to have a reaction.

For added flavor and antioxidants you can blend with green tea. Oolong Tea is very good for the skin, so you can play with that one as well.

If herbal teas do not sit well with your palate, they can be chilled and served with a sprig of mint or a dash of honey for a refreshing twist.

Now that you have started to slowly remove the toxins from the inside, it's time to start working on the outside.

Exfoliate

As we age, our metabolism begins to slow down, resulting in slower cellular movement. A buildup of cells in the body can cause sluggish blood flow throughout the veins and arteries. This can also result in cells that get stuck in little places which ultimately can result in cancer. Detoxing the internal parts of the body help remove the buildup of toxins and cells that block blood flow.

Having a sluggish metabolism not only affects the internal affairs of the body, but it occurs on the outside of the body as well. Skin is made up of a whole network of cells, and when cellular movements slow down, they also begin to collect on the outside of the body. A heavy buildup of skin cells on the surface makes us appear much older than we are, and is what most people consider dry skin.

Have you ever noticed how babies and young children have a beautiful glow to their skin? Their little bodies are hard at work doing the job that nature intended. They do not have all of the debris in their systems to slow down metabolism; their bodies are revving right along.

To give yourself a nice healthy glow, exfoliation is just the ticket to remove dead skin and prepare the body as a clean slate for your beauty products to be able to do their jobs. It does not matter how expensive or advanced your skin care is, if dead skin cells are in the way, you are wasting your time and money.

There are two ways to rid your body of those pesky dead skin cells and give yourself a glow that everyone will notice: body brushing and a sugar scrub.

Body Brushing

Body brushing has been done for centuries, and you can do this quickly each time you bathe. You can go online to places like Amazon.com for a Body Brush, or find one at your local natural food store. They are an inexpensive investment and I usually only have to replace mine every 5 years or so.

All you have to do is run the brush over your entire body before you enter your bath – it's that simple. This removes the top coat of dead skin and prepares the body for a better detox or herbal bath. I would not recommend using the body brush on your face though, it's too harsh. I have some better options for your face later in the book.

Sugar Scrub

Just like body brushing, using a sugar scrub to remove dead skin is an amazing experience. You can do both the Body Brushing and the Sugar Scrub, but it may too much on the skin to do this daily. You will know if you have over-exfoliated because your skin will feel like you have a slight sunburn.

Making your own sugar scrub is simple, and like all of the other skin care you are making, you can add whatever essential oils suit your fancy:

Tante Sophia's Sugar Scrub
- Fill a Mason Jar with ¾ cup of sugar
- Add ¼ cup of coconut oil
- Add 50 drops of Vanilla essential oil or ¼ cup of pure Vanilla extract
- Add the ingredients together slowly to ensure a good mix

You can substitute olive oil for the coconut oil if you like, and the essential oils can be switched out as you like. This is a basic scrub, and best for the beginning skin care creator.

To use the sugar scrub, stand on a towel before you enter the tub. Scoop the scrub out of the container and gently rub it all over the body and then get into the shower to rinse it off before your bath. Be careful because the floor of the tub will be slippery: Tante used to always say, "You have to suffer to be beautiful," but I don't think this is what she had in mind!

There endless options available right in your kitchen to make fantastic scrubs. Here are a few more to add to your repertoire.

Sensual Spice Body Scrub
- 3 tbsp. of olive oil
- 2 tbsp. of baby rice cereal

- 1 tsp of nutmeg
- 2 tsp of ground cloves
- ½ tsp of ground ginger
- ½ tsp ground cinnamon

Dana's Radiant Body Rub
- 2 tbsp of warm coffee grounds
- 2 tsp of sugar
- 3 tbsp of coconut oil
- 1 tsp of ground cardamom

Never underestimate what the gift of nuts can do for the body: why not try it on your skin, as well.

Nutty Pick Me Up
- Handful of cashews, finely ground
- 2 tsp of olive oil or sesame seed oil
- 2 tbsp. of honey
- 3 drops of Geranium or Grapefruit essential oil

You can also add any fruit that has gone "Beyond the Pale" into a scoop of your scrubs by mashing them into a bowl and adding them to the mixture. Rotten fruit is gift from Mother Nature and can eat dead skin instantly off of the body. Plus, it's wonderful to smell like strawberries or peaches!

Making Your Own Soap

As you begin creating your own skin care, one of the easiest things that you can do is make some special bath soap tailored just for your own needs. The added bonus of aroma makes this an even more pleasurable experience.

Making your own body and face wash is a lot of fun, and the bottles can end up being all over your house if you are not careful. If you get completely carried away you can even go so far as making your own hand soap, dish soap, and laundry soap!

No matter what you choose to do with this information, always label your creations. It wouldn't hurt you to mistakenly use your body wash on your face, but if you find something that works for you, it is important to know exactly what you put into your concoction so you can recreate it. It's oh so frustrating to make something you really love and not remember what you put into it.

The difference between one drop and to two drops sometimes can make a world of difference, and you will be upset with yourself if you cannot recall the measurements. As you become an expert kitchen scientist, you may even want to keep a journal of all your experiments. Record special memories that happen as you go along this journey as well—it is good for the soul.

Face and Body Wash

Castile   soap is an olive oil-based soap made without harsh detergents, or sulfates, and it cleanses the body naturally. It is very good for sensitive skin and even better for psoriasis and eczema. The olive oil base is a strong antioxidant which helps the body by boosting cell strength to fight disease. The addition of essential oils to the soap will further encourage the body to remain strong and fight whatever challenge is thrown at you, including stress.

- Pour 4 oz. of Castile Soap into a reusable bottle
- Add about 40 drops of the Essential Oils of your choice

Bar Soaps for Face and Body

There are many ways to make your own bar soap. My Grand'Mere always made her own soap with Lye, and it took four weeks to cure to her liking.

For our purposes here, we're going to use a melt-and-pour soap block as a base *There are lots of different kinds of glycerin based melt-and-pour soaps from olive oil or goat milk, to cocoa butter, to Aloe Vera. They are available <u>online</u> or from your local crafts or health food store.*

- 1 lb. block of melt-and-pour soap

- ~1 tsp. of Essential Oil of your choice (*to get some blending calculations you can use an online fragrance calculator if you're uncomfortable just experimenting*) <u>http://www.brambleberry.com/pages/Fragrance-Calculator.asp</u>x

- Tiny flower petals of your choice (omit these in your facial soaps)

1. Melt the soap block in a double boiler, stirring constantly.
2. Remove from heat and let the melted soap cool for a little bit.

3. Add essential oils and flower petals.

For my facial bar, I use Rose essential oil, and for my body bar, I use Lavender essential oil with little pieces of French Lavender. Using these bars of soap takes me right back to my childhood walks in Provence.

Healing Baths

As you begin to cleanse and Detox the inside of your body, add healing baths as a daily part of your beauty regimen.

Mineral Baths

Mineral Baths may sound fancy and luxurious. Really though, they are essential for good health and good skin. French women know the value of a luxurious soak – it's a balm for the soul as well as the body.

Mineral Baths are commonly prescribed by Medical Professionals to revive pain and stiffness. However, bathing in minerals is very therapeutic, especially for irritated skin.

Tantine Marguerite's Healing Bath

- ½ cup Epsom Salt

- ¼ cup Baking Soda

- 2 tbsp Sea Salt

- For sore muscles, add 8 drops of Cypress essential oil to your mixture, or for sensitive skin, add 15-20 drops of Lavender essential oil.

Fill the tub with as much water as it will hold without spilling and immerse your whole body for at least 20 minutes.

Make your bath time extra special. Light candles and turn on soothing music just to pamper yourself a bit. We women often spend most of our days taking care of everyone else, so make bath-time *your* time.

Additions to the Mineral Baths

French Clay

Clay has been used for centuries to deeply cleanse and invigorate the skin.

Add 1 cup of French Clay to your Mineral Bath
Soak for 20 minutes

Make sure that you rinse your bathtub and yourself off before leaving the bathroom: this gets a little messy and if you don't do it straight away you'll have a disaster on your hands!

Bathing with Flower Petals

Another treat to add to the bath is flower petals. A woman should have the pleasure of buying, or even better, growing flowers for herself. Fresh cut flowers are a special treat that we all love. What better way to show yourself love than bathing in the essence of flower oils. You can buy already packaged flower petals or buy flowers to enjoy in your home and wait until they wilt before using them in your bath:

- 1 medium finely-woven mesh bag
- Rubber Band or string
- 1 cup of flower petals

1. Place the flower petals into the mesh bag and ensure that the bag is securely fastened with a rubber band or string.

2. Fill the bath tub with very hot water.
3. Place the mesh bag into the tub and leave for 10 minutes. When the water cools, enter the bath.

Herbal Baths

Herbal baths are not common, but are just as easy to create as any other. It is basically the same concept as herbal teas, but on a much larger scale. Use the leaves of herbs and plants from your garden, or buy a bunch from the market to soak in the benefits of the herbs through your skin.

Patricia's Peppermint Bath

Patricia was a close friend of Maman, and I would stay with her if my parents were away. If I wasn't feeling well, she would put me in her special bath and I always seemed to feel better afterwards:

- 1 cup of Peppermint leaves stuffed into a tightly bound mesh bag
- Run a bathtub full of hot water
- Place the mesh bag into the water and let it steep for ten minutes

When I walked into the bathroom, the heady scent would open my sinuses, I'd relax in the bath, and sleep like a baby when I went to bed, no "medicine" needed!

Chamomile and Lavender can be used in the same way, and are fantastic for irritated and/or sensitive skin.

Then we have the:
Citrus Crystal Bath
- 1 tbsp. baking soda
- 4 tbsp. citric acid crystals
- 6 tbsp. baking soda
- 9 drops of essential oils

This bath is like those foaming balls you can buy to revitalize your skin.

If I have a busy day planned, I put Lemon and Lavender essential oils in this bath and it sets my day to a good start.

Bathing in Milk

Spending days playing in the lavender fields as a young girl, I would sometimes come home with overly sun-kissed skin. Maman would whisk me off to the bath while I was scolded for not protecting my skin.

A nice milk bath would fix me right up. Back then we would use powdered milk, or pureed almonds with water in a cup of milk added into the tub. Now you can buy this mix already made, so it is much easier to have this luxurious treatment. It is very soothing for eczema, rosacea, or psoriasis.

- 1 cup of organic almond or coconut milk
- 6 tbsp. of organic honey
- 10 drops of Lavender, or Chamomile, or Ylang Ylang, or a combination of all three

Soak in this luxurious bath for a total sense of wellbeing and silky skin.

Body Oils/Massage Oils

Some of us that have dry itchy skin, and scratching at it causes damage that breaks down the skin barrier, making it weak and prone to infection and disease. Using a body oil immediately after getting out of your bath or shower locks in moisture and creates a barrier to protect the skin from further dryness.

Making a body oil or a massage oil is quick and easy and you can use any varieties of oils. As always, make sure the quality of oil is the best grade that you can afford:

- Pour Almond or Jojoba oil into a 4 oz. glass bottle
- Add 15-20 drops of essential oil, depending on need
- Shake well before every use

Body oil and massage oil are basically the same thing, with the only real difference being that massage oils are generally not overly greasy, but this also depends on your skin type and how it absorbs the oil. Almond oil is the lightest oil, and a good general oil to always have on hand.

Apply your body oil while your skin is still damp; the fragrance from the essential oil will linger and your skin will feel moisturized all day long.

Lotions

All-Over Light Body Lotion

Making body lotion requires a bit more work than the other products, but is just as rewarding. You will need some organic glycerin and some unflavored gelatin to perform this little bit of magic:

- Dissolve 1 tsp. of unflavored gelatin in 1/4 cup of boiling water
- Add ¼ cup of cold water and let it sit until it thickens
- Place ½ cup of glycerin into a blender with half of the gelatin mixture.
- Add whatever you want to make this lotion your own: add essential oils for your skin type, Vitamin E, Fish Oil capsules, or whatever you think that you may need, in small quantities
- Pour into reusable glass bottles and let sit until mixture thickens

Note - You may have to add more water if it is too thick.

Adding beeswax granules to the body lotion will make a thick and luxurious product I call body butter.

Body Butter

Making a thicker form of the body lotion is an easy as melting beeswax.

You can get beeswax in sticks, beads, granules, or many different varieties.

Just melt the 1 ounce of wax slowly with the glycerin, and follow the directions above.

There are so many options available when you make your own lotion. You just have to figure out what is the best consistency for you. Applying the lotion right over the body oil will give you a reason to get out of bed every morning.

I adore roses, so I make my own rosewater, which is just like making herbal tea. Let it cool and use in place of the cold water to dissolve the gelatin.

You can also use Lavender, ground orange peels, or anything your heart desires.

Body Spray

Making body spray is as easy as filling up a bottle. I recommend getting a few small glass spray bottles for experimenting with fragrances:

Pour witch hazel in a small glass bottle fitted with a spray pump
Use up to 25 drops of Essential Oil to every 2 oz. of liquid

After introducing one of my friends to the art of hand crafted skin care, she made a body spray that I always carry in my handbag:

Emma's Afternoon Delight
- 2 oz. of freshly brewed Green Tea
- The juice of ½ of an Organic Lime
- ½ of a cucumber, sliced very thin
- 1/8 cup water, boiling

Pour boiling water over the cucumber slices and let cool
Strain the water from the cucumbers
Mix in remaining ingredients and pour into a small spray bottle.

Use all day long for a refreshing pick-me up: can be sprayed directly onto the face.

Dusting Powder

I remember growing up and hugging my aunts, and noticing how each woman had her own particular scent. It came mostly from their dusting powders, and it is that scent memory that lingers in my mind even if I can't always clearly recall their faces.

When I am feeling out of sorts and need a bit of comfort, I reach for my little jar of dusting powder.

It rarely fails to soothe my senses and set my mood right. I'm sure my husband is profoundly grateful for that little jar of powder!

Tantine's Favorite Dusting Powder
- In a clean, dry Mason Jar, place 1 cup of Cornstarch
- Add 30 drops of Vanilla Essential Oils (or any combinations of oils you like), stirring slowly after every drop using a wooden spoon
- Place the jar in a cool dry place and use a powder puff to apply to your intimate areas or any place that tends to chafe.

Caring for your Beautiful Face

The care of the skin of the face requires knowing exactly what you need.

I have yet to meet a person that has "normal" skin. The general skin types are Oily, Dry, or a Combination of the two. Finding a perfect balance is what you need to search for in regard to care of facial skin.

Read through the list of essential oils mentioned in The Foundation of Self Care and use them to create separate bottles or bars of face wash and lotion. There just a few more things that I want to discuss with you in this last lesson on skin care.

Washing the Face

I love to talk to people about skin care. I listen to them go on and on for ages about how they tried this product or that product, but nothing works for them. One of the greatest mistakes that women make when washing their face is they are not getting clean enough, especially when they wear makeup.

In the evening, after a long day, it is best if you wash your face twice and use a face brush. A face brush is similar to a body brush but softer.

- Wash the face once to get the first layer of grime, grease, and makeup off.
- Rinse that all away then cleanse one more time.
- Then, take the face brush and gently scrub the face to stimulate circulation and mildly exfoliate.

- Then rinse once more.

Correctly washing your face removes all of the build-up and the dead skin that we discussed earlier. Without cleansing the face twice, your lotions and potions cannot work the way they are intended due to the blockage of grime and dead skin.

Exfoliating with harsh face scrubs is a fatal error in judgment that you should never make. Using harsh scrubs will create little tears in the pores that will eventually turn into huge, ugly pores.

A more in-depth but gentle exfoliation can be done once monthly using very mild ingredients:

Gentle Face Scrub
- 1 tbsp. of oatmeal
- 1 tbsp. of baby rice cereal
- 1 tbsp. of Honey

Mix ingredients together in a small bowl

After cleansing, and while your face is still damp, scoop some of the mixture up and pat it onto your skin.

Gently roll the ingredients all over your face and neck.

Rinse off with warm water, apply toner, and moisturize as usual, or you can leave the scrub on for 15 minutes as a mask to soothe irritated skin, then proceed with the rinse, toner and lotion.

Toners

Regardless of your skin type you should use a Toner as it closes your pores, balances the pH of your skin, and provides a base to help your face lotion absorb evenly.

In a small misting bottle, fill ¾ full of Witch Hazel

Toner For Oily Skin
Add 10 drops of Lemon essential oil, or use the juice of ½ of an organic lemon to the witch hazel

Toner For Dry Skin
Add 10 drops of Geranium essential oil to witch hazel

You can also use green tea as a substitute for witch hazel if you prefer.

Apply the toner to freshly washed skin, and scrub it into the skin using a cotton round. Scrubbing the Toner into the skin is a more effective way of getting the ingredients into the skin's layers rather than just misting.

Your toner can also be used throughout the day as a refreshing pick-me-up.

Face Masks

Once a week, give yourself a face mask to do a deep cleanse, remove impurities, and keep the circulation flowing.

Organic Facial Mud Mask
- 1 tbsp. of organic clay

- 1 tsp. of organic apple cider vinegar, or just enough to saturate the dry powder
- 5 drops of the essential oil best suited to your skin type

1. Apply to clean face and let dry

2. After the mask has thoroughly dried, remove it with warm water.

The Clay hardens as it dries, tightening the skin, which forces out any dirt that has built up in your pores.

The Vinegar supplies much-needed Vitamin C, which triggers the body to produce the collagen that keeps you looking young and beautiful.

Yogurt Face Mask for Oily or Acne Prone Skin
If your skin is acne-prone or you have monthly breakouts, a yogurt mask is an easy way to balance everything out. Yogurt normalizes the oil production and combats bacteria.

- Simply apply ¼ to ½ cup of plain yogurt to your face.
- Let rest for 15 minutes
- Rinse

As skin ages, it begins to lose its volume and firmness. Taking care of yourself and your skin is the best thing for healthy aging. If you feel you need to tighten up a little, use:

Grand'Mere's Secret Egg Tightening Mask
2 large organic eggs

1. Crack the eggs and separate the yolks from the whites.
2. Beat the egg whites briskly until they stiffen a little.
3. Using a small pastry brush, dip the brush into the egg whites and paint all over the face, neck, and décolleté.
4. Take plastic wrap and begin wrapping the head, pulling the skin up as you go, and paying close attention to the neck area. (IMPORTANT: Leave the nose and eye area exposed.) Tuck in the loose end to secure the wrap.
5. Lie down for ten minutes and then unwrap yourself and remove the egg with warm water.

If you have someone to help you, before lying down, dip two cotton rounds in freshly brewed, but chilled, green tea.

Paint the eye area with the egg whites and place the cotton rounds over the eyes. Then cover the eyes with the plastic wrap and lie down.

This is one of my favorite tricks for feeling fresh, revitalized and renewed. Grand'Mere would be very put out if she knew I had shared her secret, so let's just keep this between you and me!

Natural Sunscreen

As much as we love the sun, too much exposure can do irreparable damage to your skin.

So the next time you're out, cover yourself with a big floppy hat, which can be a fashion statement all by itself, wear your sunglasses, and apply some sunscreen.

With so many products out there deciding what to use can be quite a struggle, so what's a natural beauty to do?

Most of the commercial products contain either zinc oxide or titanium dioxide.

Zinc oxide provides the greatest protection from the UVA and UVB rays, so it is a good idea to use this for optimal protection. Unfortunately, the cream is extremely thick and hard to rub in, so unless you want to look like a lifeguard at the beach, you need to get the powder and blend it into something easier to use.

The easiest recipe is to simply take:

- 1 cup of your body lotion
- 2 tbsp. of zinc oxide powder 2 Tablespoons of the zinc powder will give you roughly SPF 20. If you want a higher SPF, use more powder.

Mix the powder into your lotion, being careful NOT to inhale the powder.

Your Natural Skin Care Shopping List

Besides essential oils, there a number of things that you will need to begin your self-made skin care journey. Scan over this list just to get an idea of the things that you will need. Refer back to this list when you are ready to begin a project.

- Epsom Salt
- Sea Salt
- Sugar
- Corn Starch
- Oatmeal
- Cucumbers
- Organic Honey
- Organic Apple Cider Vinegar
- Olive Oil
- Vitamin E Oil or Capsules
- Jojoba Oil or Almond Oil
- Green Tea Bags
- Tea ball
- Mason Jars in a variety of sizes
- Small Glass Bottles with Lids
- Small Misting Bottles
- Nylon Mesh Ribbons
- Castile Soap
- Witch Hazel
- Beeswax Granules
- Citric Acid
- Zinc Oxide Powder

Conclusion

Thank you again for purchasing this book!

I hope it was able to open a door leading to a new way of caring for your skin.

Women are the creators in our world. Let's honor our ancestors and the women who have walked before us by taking the next step in expanding the knowledge of caring for yourself and your family naturally.

Begin researching herbs, plants, and foods that will help you better your skin and your life. Then starting adding these natural gifts of the earth to your own creations.

It has been my great pleasure to share some of the small secrets that inspire my senses and feed my spirit, and I hope they have done the same for you.

If you enjoyed this book, please take the time to share your thoughts and post a review on Amazon. It would be greatly appreciated!

A Bientot,

Elodie Lefrancois

www.ingramcontent.com/pod-product-compliance
Lightning Source LLC
Chambersburg PA
CBHW070229290526
45789CB00004B/1555